Healthy Eating For Diabetics
by James Patterson

The Most Recommended

The Essential Diabetes Cookbook

Table of Contents

1. Disclaimer

This guide, even though as precise and well timed as feasibly possible, shouldn't be regarded as medical health advice, neither as an alternative for the similar. All quality recipes and selections are supplied with all the intended knowing that information for change dimensions will likely be stringently followed, and therefore blood sugar levels can be impacted by not following personalized nutritional suggestions as instructed from your physician and/or health-care-team.

2. Healthy Eating

Healthy Eating

No foods are out of range but food options are an essential component of your diabetic issues, whether or not you have Type 1, Type 2 or an additional kind of diabetic issues.

Consuming a well-balanced diet plan - that is fresh fruit and fresh vegetables, starchy food items, non-dairy resources of proteins and dairy products - is one thing we really should all attempt to do. It is good to have a treat every now and again but the meals you select are an essential component of your diabetic issues procedure, together with prescription medication, testing and staying lively.

This info is a starting up stage to assist you eat properly when you have diabetic issues. You need to also be introduced to an authorized nutritionist for precise info, tailor-made to your requirements. For motivation on refreshing cooking suggestions

The variety of servings you will need differs from individual to individual. Your nutritionist will be in a position to guide you on how much of each individual meal group you require based on your needs and dietary objectives - e.g. weight reduction, blood sugar control or sports activities.

Fresh fruits and fresh vegetables are normally reduced in fat and unhealthy calories, whilst staying jam-packed with nutritional vitamins, mineral deposits and nutritional fibre. They can help safeguard from cardiovascular event, coronary heart illness and high blood pressure and particular types of cancer.

Aim for at the very least 5 servings. Fresh, frozen, dried and tinned fruits and fresh vegetables all add up. Strive for a combination of colours to get a broad variety of nutritional vitamins and mineral deposits as achievable.

Starchy Food Items

Breads, rice, potatoes and pasta consist of carbohydrates, which is broken down into sugar and utilized by your cellular material as energy. Select carbohydrate food that are much more slowly and gradually ingested (that is, lower GI) as these will not have an effect on your blood sugar levels as much and they will continue to keep you feeling more voluminous for a longer period. Starchy food items are normally reduced in fat and high fibre options (toasted bread and whole grain choices) will also help maintain your bowels normal, avoiding digestive system problems. Much better alternatives consist of whole wheat pasta, basmati rice, brown or wild rice, granary breads, oat-based cereals such as porridge or all-natural muesli.

Dairy Products

Milk products, cheeses and yogurt consist of calcium supplements, which will help to maintain your bones and the teeth strong. They are also a very good supply of necessary protein, but some can be excessive in fat, so opt for lower-fat options wherever you can (but look out for additional sugars in its place).

Meat, Fish, Eggs And Pulses

These food items are higher in proteins, which is required for building and replacing muscle cellular material in the entire body. They also include mineral deposits, such as iron, which are required for generating red blood cells. Omega-3 fish oils, located in oily fish such as mackerel, salmon and sardines, can assist to safeguard the cardiovascular system.

Foods High In Fat And Sugar

Theoretically, your entire body does not require any food items in this team, but consuming them in small amounts can be part of a healthy and balanced diet plan. Sweet food items and beverages will increase your blood sugar so elect for diet/light or low-calorie options. It is also well worth keeping in mind that fat is higher in unhealthy calories, so try to decrease the quantity of oil you use in your food preparation and select lower-fat options where ever possible. Minimize your consumption of unhealthy fat by exchanging butter, lard, gee and so forth with unsaturated fat such as olive, sunflower and rapeseed oils.

Set Yourself Up For Success

To set oneself up for success, think about preparing a healthy and balanced diet program as a number of tiny, manageable steps like introducing a healthy salad in your diet plan every day rather than a single huge drastic change. When your small modifications grow to be a habit, you can continue to add more healthy choices.

Eating healthily is just not about strict eating restrictions, remaining unrealistically slim, or starving yourself of the foods you love. It can save you from pills and procedures to get back your well-being. Put together much more of your dishes. Cooking much more foods in your own home will help you take control of the things you are consuming and better monitor exactly what goes into your food.

Make The Correct Modifications.

When reducing back on junk foods in your diet plan, it is crucial that you substitute all of them with healthy alternate options. Changing animal fat with fresh vegetables (for example switching butter for extra virgin olive oil) can certainly make a positive impact on your overall health. Changing animal fat for refined carbohydrate food, although (for example varying your morning meal sausage for a doughnut), will not reduce your risk for cardiovascular disease or enhance your mood.

Simplify.

Rather than becoming excessively worried about calorie counting, think about your diet plan with regards to colour, selection, and quality. Concentrate on staying away from packed and processed food and choosing much more fresh new ingredients.

Read the labels.

It's important to be aware of what's in your food as manufacturers often hide large amounts of sugar and salt in packaged food, even food claiming to be healthy.

Concentrate On Your Feelings After Consuming.

This helps promote healthy new routines and tastes. The additional wholesome foods you take in, the better you will really feel following a meal. The extra unhealthy meals you consume, the more likely you are going to really feel not comfortable, sick, or energy depleted

Drink Plenty Of Water.

Drinking water will help flush our systems of waste material and harmful toxins, however lots of people go through daily life dehydrated leading to exhaustion, very low energy, and headaches. It is popular to mistake being thirsty for food cravings, so staying properly replenished with water may also assist you create more healthy diet choices.

3. The Mouth Watering Stuffed Chicken Breast

Ingredients

Servings: 4

- **4-5-ounce boneless, skinless chicken breast halves**
- **4 water-packed canned artichoke hearts, minced**
- **¼ cup onion, minced**
- **1 teaspoon crushed dried oregano, preferably Greek**
- **salt (optional)**
- **freshly ground pepper**
- **1 tablespoon olive oil**
- **1 cup fat-free no-salt-added canned chicken broth**
- **¼ cup + 1 1/2 tablespoons fresh lemon juice**
- **4 slices lemon**
- **2 teaspoons corn-starch**
- **chopped parsley for garnish**

Directions

1. Remove all visible fat from chicken, rinse and pat dry. Season chicken with salt (if using) and pepper.

2. Place halves between 2 pieces of plastic wrap and pound with the flat side of a meat mallet until the chicken is very thin and flat.

3. Combine artichoke hearts, onion, and oregano.

4. Spoon equal amounts of the artichoke mixture into the centre of each pounded chicken breast to form a log. Roll up. Secure with a toothpick or skewers

5. Heat oil in a non-stick skillet over medium heat. Add chicken and brown evenly on all sides. If some of the stuffing drops out, don't despair. It will flavour the sauce.

6. Pour on broth and lemon juice.

7. Top chicken with lemon slices, cover and simmer until chicken is cooked through (about 15 to 20 minutes).

8. Transfer chicken to a platter, discarding toothpicks/skewers. Keep warm (covering it in foil and putting it in the oven should work well).

9. Using a fork, mix corn-starch with the remaining 1 1/2 tablespoons lemon juice. Add to skillet and stir over high heat until slightly thickened.

10. Spoon lemon sauce onto chicken. Garnish with the cooked lemon slices and parsley.

4. Chicken Noodle Soup

Ingredients

- 1 3-pound whole chicken, cut into 8 pieces
- 2 large onions: one should be peeled and quartered and one should be small diced
- 3 large carrots: one should be peeled and quartered and two should be small diced
- 3 sprigs flat-leaf parsley
- ½ teaspoon crushed dried thyme
- ½ teaspoon crushed dried marjoram
- ¼ teaspoon freshly ground pepper
- 1 quart canned no-salt, no-fat chicken broth
- 1 quart boiling water
- 6 ounces medium-wide noodles (cooked separatel
- 4 ounces button mushrooms, sliced
- ½ pound fresh spinach, well washed and large stems removed
- 2 celery stalks, diced small

Directions

1. Rinse and pat dry chicken. Place in a 5-quart or larger crockery slow cooker. Place the peeled and quirted onion, peeled and quartered carrot, and parsley around chicken pieces. Sprinkle with thyme, marjoram, and pepper.

2. Add chicken broth, cover, and cook on low for 7 to 8 hours or on high for 2 1/2 to 3 hours. When done cooking, remove and discard the onion, carrot, and parsley. Skim off and discard all surface fat from the broth.

3. Remove the chicken from broth and cool for about 10 minutes, until cool enough to handle.

4. Remove and discard the chicken skin and bones. Shred chicken.

5. Add shredded chicken back to the slow cooker and bring to a simmer. Add diced onion, diced carrots, diced celery, mushroom, and spinach. Simmer for 10 minutes.

6. Meanwhile, cook noodles according to package directions.

7. Just before serving, add cooked noodles to soup and season with salt and pepper (to taste).

5. Pork Chops with Mushrooms

Ingredients

- 1/8 ounce dried wild mushrooms, such as morels, mixed Italian etc.
- ½ cup boiling water
- cooking spray
- 4 centre-cut boneless loin pork chops, 4 ounces each, all fat removed
- freshly ground pepper
- 3 ounces fresh oyster or shiitake mushrooms
- ½ cup canned fat-free, low-sodium chicken bro
- ¼ cup dry white wine and 2 thyme sprigs

Directions

1. In a bowl, place the dried mushrooms and cover with boiling water. Follow package directions to dehydrate.

2. Drain the mushrooms. Reserve 1/4 cup of the mushroom soaking liquid.

3. Lightly coat a non-stick skillet with cooking spray. Add the chops and cook uncovered for about 5 minutes over medium heat. Turn the chops, season with pepper, reduce heat, and cook for another 8 to 9 minutes. Transfer the chops to a plate, cover, and keep warm.

4. Re-coat the same skillet with cooking spray and add both the dried and the fresh mushrooms. Sauté for 4 to 5 minutes.

5. Raise the heat, and add the chicken broth, wine, reserved mushroom soaking liquid, and thyme. Bring to a boil and reduce the liquid by half.

6. To serve, spoon the mushrooms and sauce over the pork chops.

6. Black Bean Burgers

Ingredients

- 3 spring onions, finely sliced
- 400g tin black eyed beans, drained and rinsed
- 75g granary breadcrumbs
- 100g feta cheese, crumbled
- 2 tbsp. mixed fresh herbs, chopped, eg parsley, coriander and chives
- 1 egg, beaten
- wholemeal rolls, to serve salad, red onions and tomato

Method

1. Heat half the oil in a non-stick frying pan and fry the spring onions for 1–2 minutes, until softened.

2. Place the black eyed beans in a large bowl and roughly mash. Stir in the remaining ingredients and combine well.

3. Divide the mixture into 6 and form each into patties or burgers.

4. Place on a baking sheet, brush each side with the remaining oil and chill for at least 30 minutes, or until required. Cook for 2–3 minutes on each side on a medium barbecue or grill until cooked through. Serve in a wholemeal roll and fill with green salad, tomatoes and red onion.

7. Mackerel Wraps

Ingredients

- 1 small red onion, finely chopped
- pinch salt
- juice of half a lime
- 2 tbsp. extra virgin olive oil
- ½ level tsp cumin
- pinch chili powder
- 3-4 plums, stoned and chopped
- 8-10 fresh ripe cherry tomatoes, chopped
- 1 tbsp. chopped fresh coriander
- 4 mackerel fillets
- 4 rotas or wholemeal tortillas
- 100g mixed salad leaves

Method

1. Add the onion, salt, lime juice, olive oil, cumin and chili powder to a bowl, and mix well.

2. Mix in the plums, tomatoes and coriander. Cover and set aside for 5 minutes.

3. Meanwhile, make three slits across the skin of each mackerel fillet.

4. Grill or barbecue each mackerel fillet skin side up under a grill, or skin side down on a barbecue, for around 4 minutes. This should be enough to cook the fillet right through but if not, turn it over and cook it for 1 minute on the flesh side too.

5. After warming the tortilla, add some salad leaves and a mackerel fillet. Top it with a dessert spoon of salsa and roll up.

6. Serve the rest of the salsa on the side.

8. Chicken Kebabs

Ingredients

For the marinade

- 2 tbsp. toasted coriander seeds
- 1 tbsp. toasted cumin seeds
- 4 cloves garlic, peeled
- 4cm piece ginger, roughly chopped
- 2 red chillies, de-seeded and roughly chopped
- pinch coarse salt
- freshly ground black pepper
- 1 tbsp. sun-dried tomato puree
- 3 tbsp. white wine vinegar
- 3 tbsp. extra virgin olive oil

For the kebabs

- 8 small chicken breasts, cut into 2.5-3.5cm cubes
- 4 medium courgettes, cut into 2cm thick rings
- 8 lemon or lime wedges to serve

Method

1. To make the marinade, grind the coriander and cumin seeds to a powder.

2. Pound the garlic, ginger and chillies with a pinch of salt and pepper, to a rough paste in a mortar.

3. Work in the coriander and cumin, tomato purée, vinegar, and olive oil. Mix in 2 tbsp water. Pour over the chicken pieces, and turn to coat each one.

4. Leave for at least half an hour (or up to 24 hours, covered, in the fridge).

5. Preheat the grill or bbq thoroughly. Thread the chicken pieces onto 8 long skewers or 16 small ones, alternating with courgette rings. Grill or barbecue for around 10 minutes, turning several times until browned and cooked through. Serve with lemon or lime wedges, and rice or salad.

9. Bolognese With Brown Rice

Ingredients

- **To make Healthy Bolognese, you'll need:**
- **2 onions, chopped**
- **2 carrots, grated**
- **4 cloves of garlic, finely chopped**
- **100g mushrooms, finely chopped**
- **1 stick of celery, finely diced**
- **400g lean lamb mince**
- **400g canned tomatoes, finely chopped**
- **100ml water**
- **1 tbsp. olive oil**
- **2 tbsp. tomato puree**
- **½ tsp. paprika**
- **Season with salt and pepper**
- **400g of cooked brown long grain rice (100g cooked rice per serving)**

Method

1. Sauté the onions, garlic, carrot, mushrooms and celery in the olive oil over a medium heat until softened.

2. Add the lamb and cook for 5 to10 minutes until browned.

3. Stir through the tomatoes and tomato puree cook for about 3 minutes.

4. Add the paprika and water.

5. Cover the pan and cook over a low heat for around 30 minutes until the sauce is thick and rich.

6. Season to taste and set the pan aside until ready to serve.

7. Serve immediately with the cooked brown rice.

10. Salmon With Pepper

Ingredients

1 ½ pounds fresh Salmon
½ cup white wine
¼ cup Worcestershire sauce
1 cup chicken broth, fat-free, low-sodium
¼ teaspoon salt
1 yellow onion
2 tablespoons black pepper
3 tablespoons extra virgin olive oil
4 cups fresh chopped Spinach, frozen will not work well

Preparation

1. This recipe requires at least 30 minutes of marinating time. Rinse fish and then pat dry with paper towels.

2. Cut into four 6-ounce pieces. In a resealable plastic food storage bag, combine wine, Worcestershire sauce, chicken stock and salt.

3. Peel onion and slice thinly and add to bag, along with the salmon. Refrigerate for at least 30 minutes, turning occasionally.

4. Spread black pepper on a large plate. Remove salmon, reserving marinade and onion. Press both sides of salmon into pepper to coat and set aside.

5. In a large skillet, heat olive oil over medium heat. Add onion to skillet. Cook until onion is soft, about 3 to 5 minutes. Remove with a slotted spoon and set aside.

6. Increase heat to medium-high. Place salmon, flesh side down, in the skillet and cook until crisp and browned, about 4 minutes per side.

7. When salmon is just cooked through, about 6 to 10 minutes, remove from skillet. Add spinach (washed) to skillet, and cook until limp.

8. Divide spinach equally among the serving plates. Place salmon on top. Cook marinade until reduced by half, then spoon over salmon. Serve with cooked wild rice, if desired.

11. Grilled Steak Salad

Ingredients

- **9 oz. sirloin steak**
- **1/2 tsp. salt free seasoning (such as Mrs. Dash)**
- **8 cups Mescaline salad mix**
- **1/4 red onion, thinly sliced**
- **1 cup cherry tomatoes, sliced in half lengthwise**

Instructions

1. Heat an indoor or outdoor grill. Season both sides of the steak with the salt free seasoning.

2. Grill the steak for 5-6 minutes per side or until cooked to medium well (145 degrees internal temperature) set aside to rest loosely covered with foil.

3. In a large bowl, toss together salad mix, red onion and cherry tomatoes. Divide evenly among 4 large plates.

4. Thinly slice steak and top each salad with 2 ounces of steak.
Top the steak with 3 1/2 Tbsp. of the bleu cheese salad dressing.

12. Scallops With A Twist

Ingredients

- 12 ounces dry sea scallops, cut into 1/2-inch pieces, or dry bay scallops (see Note)
- 4 teaspoons reduced-sodium tamari, or soy sauce, divided
- 4 tablespoons plus 2 teaspoons canola oil, divided
- 1 1/2 cups quinoa, rinsed well (see Tip)
- 2 teaspoons grated or minced garlic
- 3 cups water
- 1 teaspoon salt
- 1 cup trimmed and diagonally sliced snow peas, (1/2 inch thick)
- 1/3 cup rice vinegar
- 1 teaspoon toasted sesame oil
- 1 cup thinly sliced scallions
- 1/3 cup finely diced red bell pepper
- 1/4 cup finely chopped fresh cilantro, for garnish

Preparation

1. Toss scallops with 2 teaspoons tamari (or soy sauce) in a medium bowl. Set aside.

2. Place a large, high-sided skillet with a tight-fitting lid over medium heat. Add 1 tablespoon canola oil and quinoa. Cook, stirring constantly, until the quinoa begins to color, 6 to 8 minutes. Add garlic and cook, stirring, until fragrant, about 1 minute more. Add water and salt and bring to a boil. Stir once, cover and cook over medium heat until the water is absorbed, about 15 minutes. (Do not stir.) Remove from the heat and let stand, covered, for 5 minutes. Stir in snow peas, cover and let stand for 5 minutes more.

3. Meanwhile, whisk 3 tablespoons canola oil, the remaining 2 teaspoons tamari (or soy sauce), vinegar and sesame oil in a large bowl. Add the quinoa and snow peas, scallions and bell pepper; toss to combine.

4. Remove the scallops from the marinade and pat dry. Heat a large skillet over medium-high until hot enough to evaporate a drop of water upon contact. Add the remaining 2 teaspoons canola oil and cook the scallops, turning once, until golden and just firm, about 2 minutes total. Gently stir the scallops into the quinoa salad. Serve garnished with cilantro, if desired

13. Roasted Bolognese With Spaghetti

Ingredients

- 3 tbsp. olive oil

- 2 beef short ribs

- 1 red onion, quartered

- 1 onion, quartered

- 2 large carrots, cut into 4cm/2in batons

- 15 tomatoes, preferably heritage tomatoes of assorted colours

- 1 garlic bulb

- 500ml/18fl oz. beef stock

- 500g/1lb 2oz dried spaghetti

- salt and freshly ground black pepper

Preparation method

Preheat the oven to 180C/160 fan/Gas 4.

1. Heat the oil over a medium heat in a large roasting tin on the hob. Add the short ribs and fry for 3-4 minutes on all sides, or until browned all over. Add the onions and carrots, and then transfer to the oven for 45 minutes.

2. After 45 minutes, tuck the tomatoes and the whole garlic bulb into the roasting tin, pour in the beef stock and continue to cook for a further hour.

3. Towards the end of the cooking time, cook the spaghetti according to the packet instructions, then drain well and set aside.

4. Remove the beef ribs from the roasting tin and set aside on a chopping board to rest.

5. Squeeze the garlic cloves from their skins into the roasting tin. Using a slotted spoon or fork, lightly squash the tomatoes and mix them and the garlic into the sauce.

6. slide the short-rib meat off the bones and cut it into strips. Return the meat to the roasting tin.

7. Stir in the cooked pasta, then season with salt and freshly ground black pepper, and serve.

14. Stir-Fry

Ingredients

- 2 tbsp. sunflower oil
- 4 spring onions, cut into 4cm/1½in lengths
- 1 garlic clove, crushed
- piece fresh root ginger, about 1cm/½in, peeled and grated
- 1 carrot, cut into matchsticks
- 1 red pepper, cut into thick matchsticks
- 100g/3½oz baby sweetcorn, halved
- 1 courgette, cut into thick matchsticks
- 150g/5½oz sugar-snap peas or mange tout, trimmed
- 2 tbsp. hoisin sauce
- 2 tbsp. low-salt soy sauce

Preparation method

1. Heat a wok on a high heat and add the sunflower oil. Add the spring onions; garlic, ginger and stir-fry for 1 minute, then reduce the heat. Take care to not brown the vegetables.

2. Add the carrot, red pepper and baby sweetcorn and stir-fry for 2 minutes. Add the courgette and sugar snap peas and stir-fry for a further 3 minutes. Toss the ingredients from the centre to the side of the wok using a wooden spatula. Do not overcrowd the wok and keep the ingredients moving.

3. Add 1 tablespoon water, hoisin and soy sauce and cook over a high heat for a further 2 minutes or until all the vegetables are cooked but not too soft. Serve with noodles or rice.

15. Green Pasta Salad

Ingredients

- **250g ouzo**
- **4tbsp extra virgin olive oil**
- **200g green beans**
- **3 medium courgettes, trimmed**
- **5 spring onions, finely chopped**
- **150g pitted green olives, sliced**
- **3tbsp small (non peril) capers**
- **zest and juice of 1 lemon**
- **2 avocados, chopped**
- **5tbsp chopped flat-leaf parsley**

Preparation

1. Cook the pasta in plenty of boiling salted water until tender. Drain, run it under cold water, toss away any excess water then add the oil and stir well. Bring a pan of salted water to the boil and blanch the beans for 2 minutes. Run under cold water, and then chop into small pieces.

2. Using a ribbon peeler, cut the courgettes into ribbons.

3. Combine all the ingredients together, season well with salt and pepper and serve.

16. Chili Sea Bass

Ingredients

- 1 x 1kg whole sea bass, gutted and scaled
- ½ bunch fresh coriander, roughly chopped
- 2 red chillies, finely chopped
- 1 tbsp. cumin seeds, toasted
- 2 tbsp. extra-virgin olive oil
- sea salt

For the dressing

- juice of 2 limes
- 1 tsp unrefined light muscovado sugar
- 1 tsp fish sauce
- 2 tbsp. olive oil

Preparation

Preheat the oven to 190°C/gas 5

1. Clean the sea bass, wiping it inside and out with kitchen paper

2. Use a sharp knife to gently score the fish with 3–4 diagonal cuts on both sides. Stuff the inside of the fish with the fresh coriander

3. Mix together the chillies, cumin seeds, olive oil and salt and rub this mixture all over the outside of the fish. Place the fish on a baking tray and bake in the oven for about 30 minutes. The skin should crisp up nicely as the fish is not covered

4. Check if the fish is cooked – the flesh should be opaque and feel firm to the touch. Return to the oven for a further 5 minutes if necessary. Meanwhile, whisk together the dressing ingredients. Once the fish is cooked, remove the fillets using two spoons and then drizzle a little dressing over each portion

17. Chili And Grilled Mackerel

Ingredients

- 1tsp crushed black peppercorns
- 2tsp ground coriander
- 1tbsp finely grated lemon zest
- 4 oranges
- 1 red chili, de-seeded and finely chopped
- 8 x 150g mackerel fillets (not smoked)
- 2tbsp chopped coriander
- 110g watercress
- 1 small red onion, peeled and thinly sliced

Method

1. Preheat the grill to high. Mix the black peppercorns, ground coriander and lemon zest together in a bowl. Grate the zest from half an orange and stir into the coriander mixture with half the chopped red chili.

2. Lightly cut the skin of the mackerel and press the mixture onto the fish. Place the mackerel on a grill rack and grill, skin-side up, for 5 minutes or until crisp and cooked through. Sprinkle with the chopped coriander.

3. Meanwhile, segment the oranges. First slice the top and bottom off each orange, then cut away the peel and any white pith using a small, sharp knife. Cut down either side of each segment to release it.

4. Divide the watercress between four plates and scatter with the orange segments, sliced red onion and remaining chili. Top with the grilled mackerel and serve immediately.

18. Baked Chili Salmon

Ingredients

- **1 pack of skinless boneless salmon fillets**
- **1/2 red chili, de-seeded and finely chopped**
- **1 tomato, sliced**
- **3 tablespoons of basil pesto**

Method

1. Preheat oven to 190°C/375°F/Gas Mark 5.

2. Place the fillets in a lightly oiled backing dish. Cover the fillets in the pesto, sprinkle with chilli and layer the sliced tomato on top. This can be prepared in advance and kept in the fridge.

3. Bake in the oven for 20-25 minutes, until the salmon is cooked through.

4. Serve with a crisp green salad.

19. Roasted Carrots

Ingredients

- 700g carrots, cut on a diagonal into 3-inch-long pieces, halved lengthwise
- 120ml low-sodium vegetable or chicken broth
- 4 teaspoons olive oil
- Salt and freshly ground black pepper
- 2 tbsp. chopped mint
- 2 tbsp. chopped parsley
- 2 teaspoons fresh lemon juice
- 1/2 teaspoon finely grated lemon zest

Method

1. Place the carrots, broth and 1 teaspoon of the oil in a large pan and bring to a boil over medium-high heat. Cover, reduce the heat to medium and continue to cook until the carrots are tender, 12 to 14 minutes. Uncover and cook, stirring, until the liquid has evaporated and the carrots are lightly browned, another 2 to 3 minutes. Season with 1/4 teaspoon salt and 1/4 teaspoon pepper.

2. Meanwhile, combine the mint, parsley, juice, zest and remaining 3 teaspoons oil in a small dish. Sprinkle with salt and pepper. Toss the warm carrots with the herb mixture.

20. Green Smoothie

Ingredients

- 2 large avocados, stone removed and skin discarded
- 180g fresh baby spinach leaves
- 1 green apple
- 1 kiwi
- 500ml water
- 1 tsp agave nectar
- Handful fresh basil, plus more for garnishing

Method

1. Place all the ingredients in a high-powered blender and blend until smooth.

2. Pour into Kilned mugs and decorate with extra basil.

21. Thai Salad

Ingredients

Serves: 10

- 175g vermicelli pasta
- 110g shredded cabbage
- 2 large carrots, shredded
- 1/2 small green pepper, chopped
- 1/2 small red pepper, chopped
- 1/2 small yellow pepper, chopped
- 15g fresh coriander, chopped
- 1/2 bunch fresh spring onions, chopped
- 40g chopped peanuts
- 1 tablespoon toasted black sesame seeds
- 125g cooked prawns
- 2 tablespoons peanut butter
- 1 tablespoon tahini
- 2 tablespoons rice wine vinegar
- 2 tablespoons sweet chilli sauce
- 2 1/2 tablespoons soy sauce
- 1/2 teaspoon sesame oil
- 1/2 teaspoon dark brown sugar
- 1/2 teaspoon garlic powder
- 1/2 teaspoon salt
- 1/2 teaspoon ground black pepper

Method

1. Bring a large pot of lightly salted water to the boil. Break pasta into small pieces and add to boiling water; cook for 8 to 10 minutes or until al dente; drain. In a large bowl, toss together the pasta, cabbage, carrots, green, red and yellow peppers, 1/2 of the coriander, 1/2 of the onions and prawns.

2. In a small bowl, stir together the peanut butter, tahini, rice wine vinegar and sweet chilli sauce. Season with soy sauce, sesame oil, brown sugar, garlic powder, salt and pepper. Ten minutes before serving, toss the sauce with the cabbage mixture until evenly coated. Garnish with remaining coriander, spring onions, peanuts and black sesame seeds.

22. Spiced Shrimp

Ingredients

- **1 lb.   peeled and deveined large shrimp**
- **1 garlic clove, finely minced**
- **1/2 tsp. smoked paprika**
- **1/2 tsp. chili powder**
- **1 Tbsp. olive oil, divided**
- **2 tsp. fresh lemon juice**

Directions

1. Preheat the oven to 425 degrees. Bring the water for the pasta to boiling. Meanwhile, prepare the asparagus and place it on a foil-lined baking sheet in the oven to roast for about 10 minutes. Add the pasta to the boiling water. Prepare Simply Spiced Shrimp. Drain the pasta. Plate the pasta, shrimp, and asparagus. Slice the apple and sprinkle with cinnamon. Serve and enjoy!

2. In a bowl, mix together the shrimp, garlic, paprika, and chili powder, tossing to coat. Add 1 tsp. of the olive oil and the lemon juice. Let stand 3 minutes.

3. In a large skillet, heat the remaining 2 tsp. oil over medium-high heat. Add the shrimp and sauté on both sides for a total of 3 minutes, or until the shrimp is just opaque and cooked through.

23. Stuffed Sweet Potatoes

Ingredients

- **4 medium sweet potatoes**
- **3 cups broccoli florets**
- **4 tsp trans-fat-free margarine**
- **4 Tbsp. slivered almonds, toasted**

Instructions

1. Pierce each sweet potato with a fork in a few spots. Arrange the potatoes on a microwave-safe plate and microwave until soft, about 12 minutes.

2. Place 3/4 to 1 inch of water in a saucepan with a steamer and bring to a boil. (If you don't have a steamer, you can simply put the broccoli directly into 1 inch of boiling water.) Add the broccoli to the steamer and cover; reduce the heat to medium and let it cook for 6 minutes.

3. Using a knife slit each sweet potato in half and pinch the sides to open it up. Fill each sweet potato with 1 tsp margarine, 2/3 cup broccoli and 1 tbsp. toasted almonds.

24. Beef & Potato Casserole

Ingredients

- 1 1/2 pounds broccoli, cut into 1-inch florets (about 6 cups)
- 2 tablespoons canola oil, divided
- 1 1/2 pounds 95%-lean ground beef
- 1 large onion, chopped
- 2 tablespoons Worcestershire sauce
- 1 teaspoon garlic powder
- 1 1/4 teaspoons salt, divided
- 4 cups low-fat milk
- 1/3 cup corn-starch
- 2 cups shredded sharp Cheddar cheese, preferably orange
- 1/4 teaspoon ground turmeric
- 4 cups frozen hash-brown or precooked shredded potatoes (see Note)
- 1 large egg, lightly beaten
- 1/2 teaspoon freshly ground pepper
- Canola or olive oil cooking spray
- 1/4 teaspoon Hungarian paprika, preferably hot

Preparation

1. Preheat oven to 450°F.

2. Toss broccoli with 1 tablespoon oil in a large bowl. Spread out on a baking sheet and roast, stirring once halfway though, until just soft and browned in spots, about 15 minutes.

3. Meanwhile, heat the remaining 1 tablespoon oil in a large skillet over medium heat. Add beef and onion and cook, breaking up the beef with a wooden spoon, until the beef is browned and the onion is softened, 10 to 12 minutes. Stir in Worcestershire, garlic powder and 1/4 teaspoon salt. Set aside.

4. Whisk milk and corn-starch in a large saucepan. Bring to a boil over medium-high heat, whisking often, until bubbling and thickened enough to coat the back of a spoon, 6 to 8 minutes total. Remove from the heat and stir in Cheddar, 3/4 teaspoon salt and turmeric until the cheese is melted.

5. Spread the beef mixture in a 9-by-13-inch (or similar 3-quart) baking dish. Top with the broccoli and pour the cheese sauce evenly over the top.

6. Combine potatoes, egg, pepper and the remaining 1/4 teaspoon salt in a medium bowl. Sprinkle evenly over the casserole. Coat the top with cooking spray.

7. Bake the casserole until it is bubbling and the potatoes are beginning to brown, about 40 minutes. Sprinkle with paprika. Let stand for 10 minutes before serving.

The Most Recommended

The Essential Diabetes Cookbook
Beat and Reverse Your Type 2 Diabetes Now!
Healthy Eating for Diabetes